MULTI-SYSTEMIC SCLEROSIS DIET HANDBOOK

A COMPLETE DIET PLAN FOR THOSE WITH MULTI-SYSTEMIC SCLEROSIS

DR. JESSIE PEAKE

Table of Contents

CHAPTER ONE

Multi-systemic sclerosis

Foods to eat if you have MS

When the body's immune system attacks the brain and spinal cord in the wrong place, multiple sclerosis (MS) occurs. The disease of multiple sclerosis (MS) has no known cure, but there are some treatments and dietary choices that may help some people cope with the illness.

Damage to the myelin sheath that covers nerve fibers occurs as a result of multiple sclerosis. Electrical signals can no longer be transmitted through nerves due to this.

Multiple Sclerosis (MS) sufferers experience symptoms that fluctuate from time to time. Symptom flare-ups, or relapses, and periods of remission are common in people with mental health issues. The symptoms of other forms of MS, such as those that progress, worsen over time.

A person's symptoms and ability to cope with MS are the primary goals of MS treatment. An MS patient's overall health can be improved by eating a well-balanced diet.

It is possible to reduce the number of relapses, the risk of health complications, and improve one's quality of life by learning about the role of the diet in MS and making changes.

MS and a healthy diet go hand in hand.

Pin it to Pinterest

When the immune system attacks the nervous system, it results in multiple sclerosis (MS).

MS and diet may be linked in a variety of ways, including:

gut bacteria's role in immune disorders

- deficiency of vitamins

that certain nutrients have a protective effect on the nervous system

- the health benefits of a well-balanced, nutritious diet

Consumable foodstuffs

The immune system, nerves, and body of people with multiple sclerosis (MS) may benefit from certain foods.

Prebiotics and probiotics are both important components of a healthy digestive system.

The immune system may be affected by changes in gut health. Gut health has been linked to a wide range of health issues, according to studies.

There are many types of microorganisms that live in our digestive system, and the intestinal flora, or gut flora, is the most complex. Bacteria make up the majority of these microorganisms in humans.

Food and nutrients must be broken down by these bacteria in order for the immune system to function properly. A well-balanced diet that includes plenty of fiber helps to maintain a healthy microbiome in the digestive tract.

Probiotics, for example, may be beneficial for people with multiple sclerosis, according to a study published in 2016.

Probiotics

Supplements and a variety of fermented foods contain

probiotic bacteria. Lactobacillus, a type of beneficial bacteria, can be found in the following:

• yogurt

• kefir

• kimchi

• sauerkraut

• kombucha, a type of tea that has been fermented

Prebiotics

After introducing good bacteria to the digestive system, it is critical to provide them with food. Prebiotics are foods that support the growth of probiotic bacteria. There are prebiotic dietary fibers.

Prebiotic fiber can be found in the following foods in adequate amounts:

- artichokes

- garlic

- leeks

- asparagus

- onions

- chicory

Fiber

Many plant-based foods contain high levels of fiber, such as:

- fruits
- vegetabl
- Seeds and nuts

lentils, peas, and other legumes

grains in their natural state.

CHAPTER TWO

People with multiple sclerosis (MS) may benefit from consuming these products. A diet high in fiber has numerous benefits for the body, including:

• feeding the good bacteria in the gut

promoting regular bowel movements

control of hypertension

maintaining cardiovascular health by lowering cholesterol levels

by increasing satiety and decreasing appetite, it can help people lose weight.

Certain types of heart disease may be more common in people with MS. These risks may not be reduced by dietary measures, but a well-balanced diet is good for overall heart health.

The D-complex vitamin

MS patients may benefit especially from vitamin D, which is essential for everyone.

Those with high vitamin D levels appear to be less likely to develop multiple sclerosis, according to the National Institute of Neurological Disorders and StrokeTrusted Source.

Bone health necessitates adequate intake of vitamin D. Low bone density and osteoporosis may be more common in MS patients, especially if they have difficulty moving around. Vitamin D may play a role in preventing this.

The majority of one's vitamin D intake comes from the sun, but it can also be obtained through the following foods:

• fatty seafood

dairy products that have been fortified

cereals, yogurt and orange juice that are fortified with vitamin C

Hepatobiliary organs of cattle

in addition to the egg whites

According to a review published in 2017, further research is needed to confirm a link between low vitamin D levels and MS.

Biotin

Biotin is a type of vitamin B that is found in many foods. It can be found in a wide variety of foods, but biotin-rich foods include:

• eggs

Hepatobiliary organs of cattle

* almonds

* spinach

* broccoli

sourdough bread

People with progressive MS may benefit from taking a high dose of biotin (between 100 and 600 milligrams per day), according to findings from small studies.

Biotin supplementation is still under investigation, but people who eat a well-balanced diet are more likely to get enough of this vitamin.

Omega-3 fatty acids, also called polyunsaturated fatty acids

Polyunsaturated fatty acids (PUFAs) have been shown to support a healthy body and to control inflammation in animal studies.

PUFA intake has been linked to an increased risk of multiple sclerosis (MS) in a 2017 study, for example.

PUFAs appear to improve a wide range of bodily functions, from heart health to mental sharpness. Salmon and mackerel, as well as some plant-based oils, contain polyunsaturated fatty acids (PUFAs).

Antioxidants

Polyphenols, which are found in a wide variety of plant-based foods, have antioxidant and anti-inflammatory properties.

Polyphenols may be beneficial for people with multiple sclerosis because of their ability to protect cells from oxidative stress.

Polyphenols can be found in foods like:

- fruits

- vegetables

- spices

- cereals

- legumes

- herbs

- tea

Researchers have linked oxidative stress to the development of several chronic conditions, including neurological and cardiovascular disease, and believe that antioxidants can help prevent it.

Visit our nutrition hub for even more evidence-based information.

Foods to steer clear of.

MS sufferers should avoid certain foods.

foods high in trans fats and refined carbohydrates

Especially if they contain a high concentration of the following substances:

hydrogenated oils and triglycerides; saturated fats; trans fats;

• the addition of sodium

• the addition of sugar

Sodium

According to a study published in 2015, people with MS who consume moderate to high amounts of sodium are more likely to relapse or develop a new lesion.

Inflammation can occur as a result of this. Diets rich in antioxidant-rich fresh fruits and vegetables can help to reduce inflammation.

It's important to know what to avoid.

Those with multiple sclerosis (MS) could benefit from avoiding:

The consumption of sugar-sweetened beverages, such as soda and energy drinks

Too much processed meat, such as hot dogs and hamburger patties.

CHAPTER THREE

French fries, potato chips, and other deep-fried snacks

Frozen pizzas and other prepared foods that have undergone extensive processing

• Margarine and shortening contain trans fats.

Loss of weight

There is evidence that obesity in childhood and adolescence may raise the risk of developing multiple sclerosis. Obesity, according to the review's authors, may have an impact on how quickly the disease develops.

As a result, a person with multiple sclerosis (MS) who loses mobility or has difficulty moving may gain weight.

Controlling one's eating habits to maintain a healthy weight may also help to slow the progression of MS symptoms. Changing one's diet may improve one's overall health and well-being while also lowering one's risk of developing other ailments, such as cardiovascular disease.

Dieters must make sure they get all the nutrients they need each day, no matter what kind of diet they're on. Replacement of lost nutrients is essential for those who restrict their diet to a specific food or food group.

a diet free of gluten

MS and gluten sensitivity have not been linked in research.

However, celiac disease, which prevents the body from tolerating gluten, may be more common in people with MS than in the general population. People with multiple sclerosis may thus benefit from cutting out gluten.

Wheat, rye, and barley all contain gluten, which is a type of protein. Foods containing these grains should be avoided by those who avoid gluten.

Gluten-containing foods include:

In addition to bread and baked goods, wheat products include

Soups and salad dressings that are already prepared

Malt, soups, beer and brewer's yeast are all examples of products made from barley.

In bread and cereals, rye is an important ingredient.

Fiber, which is found in whole grains, may be missing from the diets of those who avoid gluten.

So they should eat plenty of fresh vegetables, fruits, nuts, seeds and pulses in order to increase their fiber intake, which will help them feel fuller longer.

A doctor should be consulted before embarking on a gluten-free diet.

The Paleolithic way of eating

Paleo or Paleolithic diet adherents believe that the human body has not evolved to digest the modern diet's abundance of highly processed foods.

Foods that hunter-gatherers may have eaten are incorporated into the diet. The first step is to stick to whole, unprocessed foods like meat and vegetables rather than processed ones.

Researchers found that a modified Paleolithic diet improved fatigue severity and quality of life for people with relapsing-remitting multiple sclerosis in a 2017 pilot study. Researchers conclude that further studies are needed to fully evaluate the benefits of a paleo diet for people with multiple sclerosis (MS).

Diet plan Wahls

It is a variation of the paleo diet known as the Wahls diet, or Wahls protocol. Dr. Terry Wahls designed the strategy with MS patients in mind.

The Wahls diet is similar to the paleo diet in that it emphasizes whole, minimally processed foods with a high concentration of nutrients. Green, leafy and sulfur-rich vegetables, brightly colored fruits, and minimally processed animal proteins are the staples of the Wahls diet.

Studies of a more modest scope

The Wahls diet has been linked to a reduction in MS symptoms by a reputable source. However, in order to fully examine the diet's efficacy, larger randomized studies with better controls are required.

CHAPTER FOUR

The swanky diet

During the 1950s, doctors created the Swank diet as an MS treatment.

It recommends limiting daily unsaturated fat intake to 20–50 grams and restricting daily saturated fat intake to 15 g.

Participants on this plan:

no processed foods or dairy fats can be consumed

red meat is banned for the first year

As many white fish and shellfish as they want

fruits and vegetables should be consumed in equal amounts every day.

• pasta should be made of whole grain

every day, you should be taking cod liver oil and multivitamins

The diet is viewed as dated by some, but it has been found to be beneficial by other people.

Risks include, for example,

Folic acid and vitamins A, C, and E deficiency in Trusted Source.

Compared to each other, how do the diets stack up?

The National Multiple Sclerosis Society conducted a review of various diets and their effects on MS in 2015.

It's not clear which diet is best, according to the review authors, who acknowledge that most diets restrict or exclude the same foods.

• are subjected to a high degree of processing.

saturate fat content is high

Glycemic index: foods that are high in sugar

Modifications in way of life

An MS patient's diet should focus on boosting their immune system.

Consider making the following changes, which may be helpful:

in order to raise vitamin D levels by increasing exposure to the sun

As part of a healthy lifestyle, it is important to engage in physical activity on a regular basis.

- Avoiding exposure to secondhand smoke and quitting smoking if necessary

A doctor's advice should be sought before making significant dietary or lifestyle changes.

Outlook

When MS attacks the nervous system, it can set off a cascade of health problems, both immediate and long-term. It is a long-term condition that can either improve or worsen.

A mild tingling sensation may be all that is felt by some people, while others lose the ability to walk or speak. There are, however, many MS patients who remain mobile and have the same life expectancies as their peers without the disease.

Summary

People with MS can benefit from a healthy diet, and certain dietary adjustments may slow the progression of the disease or prevent certain symptoms.

Overall, a nutritious diet can improve one's health and well-being while also reducing the risk of health problems like cardiovascular disease.

MS symptoms and associated complications may be better managed and even reduced with the use of a variety of special diets. A person should consult a doctor before making any dietary changes, and more research is needed to determine the efficacy of these diets.

THE END